Keto Air Fryer Cooking Plan

A Quick and Easy Plan for Beginners

Lydia Gorman

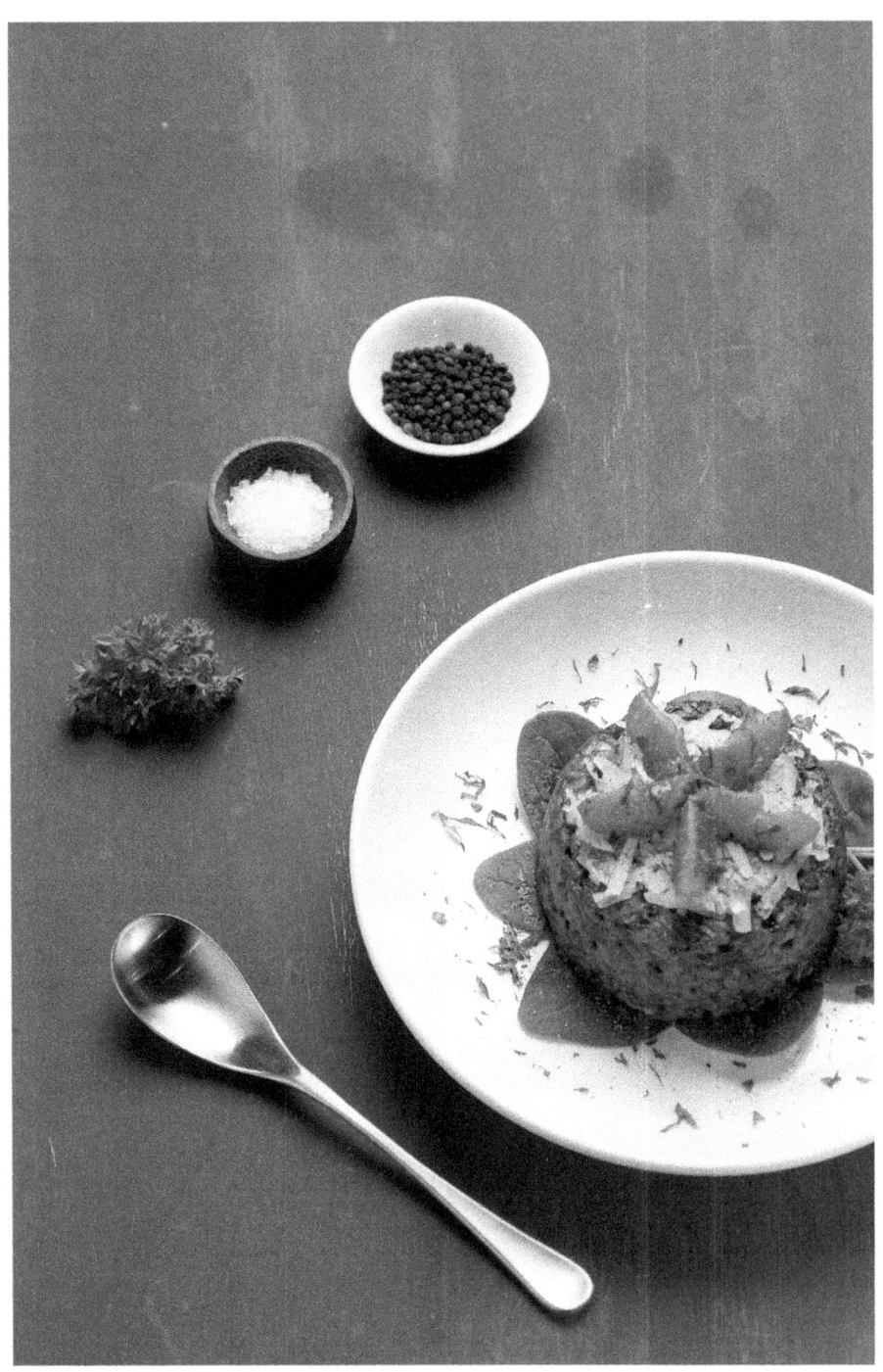

© Copyright 2020 All rights reserved.

The following Book is reproduced below with the goal of providing information that is as accurate and reliable as possible. Regardless, purchasing this Book can be seen as consent to the fact that both the publisher and the author of this book are in no way experts on the topics discussed within and that any recommendations or suggestions that are made herein are for entertainment purposes only. Professionals should be consulted as needed prior to undertaking any of the action endorsed herein.

This declaration is deemed fair and valid by both the American Bar Association and the Committee of Publishers Association and is legally binding throughout the United States.

Furthermore, the transmission, duplication, or reproduction of any of the following work including specific information will be considered an illegal act irrespective of

if it is done electronically or in print. This extends to creating a secondary or tertiary copy of the work or a recorded copy and is only allowed with the express written consent from the Publisher. All additional right reserved.

The information in the following pages is broadly considered a truthful and accurate account of facts and as such, any inattention, use, or misuse of the information in question by the reader will render any resulting actions solely under their purview. There are no scenarios in which the publisher or the original author of this work can be in any fashion deemed liable for any hardship or damages that may befall them after undertaking information described herein.

Additionally, the information in the following pages is intended only for informational purposes and should thus be thought of as universal. As befitting its nature, it is presented without assurance regarding its prolonged validity or interim quality. Trademarks that are mentioned are done without written consent and can in no way be considered an endorsement from the trademark holder.

Table of Contents

EASY TOASTED NUTS 10

CINNAMON PEAR CHIPS 11

CRUNCHY ROASTED CHICKPEAS... 12

BAKED CHEESE CRISPS 15

SOUTHERN CHEESE STRAWS.. 16

CRUNCHY BROCCOLI FRIES 18

BEER BATTERED VIDALIA RINGS 20

AVOCADO FRIES WITH LIME SAUCE... 22

KALE CHIPS WITH TAHINI SAUCE... 24

THYME-ROASTED SWEET POTATOES 26

COCKTAIL CRANBERRY MEATBALLS 29

TERIYAKI CHICKEN DRUMETTES... 31

BLUE CHEESY POTATO WEDGES 34

YAKITORI JAPANESE CHICKEN SKEWERS 35

PECORINO ROMANO MEATBALLS 37

ROMANO CHEESE AND BROCCOLI BALLS.................................... 39

PAPRIKA AND CHEESE FRENCH FRIES 41

HOT CHEESY MUSHROOMS BITES 43

PORK CRACKLING WITH SRIRACHA DIP 45

CHEESY POTATO PUFFS 47

PEPPER AND BACON MINI SKEWERS 49

WONTON SAUSAGE APPETIZERS 50

SOUTHWESTERN CAPRESE BITES 52

SALMON, CHEESE AND CUCUMBER BITES 54

MINT PLANTAIN BITES 57

PAPRIKA POTATO CHIPS 59

STICKY GLAZED WINGS 61

ASIAN TWIST CHICKEN WINGS 63

BEER-BATTERED VIDALIA ONION RINGS 65

COCONUT BANANA CHIPS 67

EGGPLANT PARM CHIPS 69

MEXICAN CRUNCHY CHEESE STRAWS 70

GREEK-STYLE DEVILED EGGS 73

PUERTO RICAN TOSTONES 75

GREEN BEAN CRISPS 76

QUICK AND EASY POPCORN 78

HOMEMADE RANCH TATER TOTS 80

BARBECUE LITTLE SMOKIES 82

BABY CARROTS WITH ASIAN FLAIR 83

GREEK-STYLE SQUASH CHIPS 85

CAJUN CHEESE STICKS 87

KALE CHIPS WITH WHITE HORSERADISH MAYO 89

MEXICAN CHEESY ZUCCHINI BITES 91

HOMEMADE APPLE CHIPS 93

EASY AND DELICIOUS PIZZA PUFFS 95

PARTY GREEK KEFTEDES 97

THREE MEAT CHEESY OMELET 99

ORANGE CREAMY CUPCAKES 101

AVOCADO TEMPURA 103

BLUEBERRY OAT BARS 104

Introduction

What's the difference between an air fryer and deep fryer? Air fryers bake food at a high temperature with a high-powered fan, while deep fryers cook food in a vat of oil that has been heated up to a specific temperature. Both cook food quickly, but an air fryer requires practically zero preheat time while a deep fryer can take upwards of 10 minutes. Air fryers also require little to no oil and deep fryers require a lot that absorb into the food. Food comes out crispy and juicy in both appliances, but don't taste the same, usually because deep fried foods are coated in batter that cook differently in an air fryer vs a deep fryer. Battered foods needs to be sprayed with oil before cooking in an air fryer to help them color and get crispy, while the hot oil soaks into the batter in a deep fryer. Flour-based batters and wet batters don't cook well in an air fryer, but they come out very well in a deep fryer.

The ketogenic diet is one such example. The diet calls for a very small number of carbs to be eaten. This means food such as rice, pasta, and other starchy vegetables like potatoes are off the menu. Even relaxed versions of the keto diet minimize carbs to a large extent and this compromises the goals of many dieters. They end up having to exert large amounts of willpower to follow the diet. This doesn't do them any favors since willpower is like a muscle. At some point, it tires and this is when the dieter goes right back to their old pattern of eating. I have personal experience with this. In terms of health benefits, the keto diet offers the most. The reduction of carbs forces your body to mobilize fat and this results in automatic fat loss and better health.

Feel free to mix and match the recipes you see in here and play around with them. Eating is supposed to be fun! Unfortunately, we've associated fun eating with unhealthy food. This doesn't have to be the case. The air fryer, combined with the Mediterranean diet, will make your mealtimes fun-filled again and full of taste. There's no grease and messy cleanups to deal with anymore. Are you excited yet?

You should be! You're about to embark on a journey full of air fried goodness!

Easy Toasted Nuts

Prep + Cook Time: 10 minutes

4 Servings

INGREDIENTS

½ cup pecans

1 cup almonds

2 tablespoons egg white

1 tablespoon granulated sugar

A pinch of coarse sea salt

DIRECTIONS

Toss the pecans and almonds with the egg white, granulated sugar and salt until well coated.

Transfer the pecans and almonds to the Air Fryer cooking basket.

Roast the pecans and almonds at 360 degrees F for about 6 to 7 minutes, shaking the basket once or twice.

Taste and adjust seasonings. Enjoy!

Cinnamon Pear Chips

Prep + Cook Time: 10 minutes

2 Servings

INGREDIENTS

1 large pear, cored and sliced

1 teaspoon apple pie spice blend

1 teaspoon coconut oil

1 teaspoon honey

DIRECTIONS

Toss the pear slices with the spice blend, coconut oil and honey.

Then, place the pear slices in the Air Fryer cooking basket and cook at 360 degrees F for about 8 minutes.

Shake the basket once or twice to ensure even cooking.

Pear chips will crisp up as it cools.

Enjoy!

Crunchy Roasted Chickpeas

Prep + Cook Time: 20 minutes

2 Servings

INGREDIENTS

1 tablespoon extra-virgin olive oil

8 ounces can chickpeas, drained

½ teaspoon smoked paprika

½ teaspoon ground cumin

½ teaspoon garlic powder

Sea salt, to taste

DIRECTIONS

Drizzle olive oil over the drained chickpeas and transfer them to the Air Fryer cooking basket.

Cook your chickpeas in the preheated Air Fryer at 395 degrees F for 13 minutes.

Turn your Air Fryer to 350 degrees F and cook an additional 6 minutes.

Toss the warm chickpeas with smoked paprika, cumin, garlic and salt.

Enjoy!

Baked Cheese Crisps

Prep + Cook Time: 15 minutes

4 Servings

INGREDIENTS

½ cup Parmesan cheese, shredded

1 cup Cheddar cheese, shredded

1 teaspoon Italian seasoning

½ cup marinara sauce

DIRECTIONS

Start by preheating your Air Fryer to 350 degrees F.

Place a piece of parchment paper in the cooking basket.

Mix the cheese with the Italian seasoning.

Add about 1 tablespoon of the cheese mixture per crisp to the basket, making sure they are not touching.

Bake for 6 minutes or until browned to your liking.

Work in batches and place them on a large tray to cool slightly.

Serve with the marinara sauce. Enjoy!

Southern Cheese Straws

Prep + Cook Time: 30 minutes

6 Servings

INGREDIENTS

1 cup all-purpose flour

Sea salt and ground black pepper, to taste

¼ teaspoon smoked paprika

½ teaspoon celery seeds

4 ounces mature Cheddar, cold, freshly grated

1 sticks butter

DIRECTIONS

Start by preheating your air Fryer to 330 degrees F.

Line the Air Fryer basket with parchment paper.

In a mixing bowl, thoroughly combine the flour, salt, black pepper, paprika, and celery seeds.

Then, combine the cheese and butter in the bowl of a stand mixer.

Slowly stir in the flour mixture and mix to combine well.

Then, pack the dough into a cookie press fitted with a star disk.

Pipe the long ribbons of dough across the parchment paper.

Then cut into six-inch lengths.

Bake in the preheated Air Fryer for 15 minutes.

Repeat with the remaining dough.

Let the cheese straws cool on a rack.

You can store them between sheets of parchment in an airtight container.

Enjoy!

Crunchy Broccoli Fries

Prep + Cook Time: 15 minutes

4 Servings

INGREDIENTS

1 pound broccoli florets

½ teaspoon onion powder

1 teaspoon granulated garlic

½ teaspoon cayenne pepper

Sea salt and ground black pepper, to taste

2 tablespoons sesame oil

4 tablespoons parmesan cheese, preferably freshly grated

DIRECTIONS

Start by preheating the Air Fryer to 400 degrees F.

Blanch the broccoli in salted boiling water until al dente, about 3 to 4 minutes.

Drain well and transfer to the lightly greased Air Fryer basket.

Add the onion powder, garlic, cayenne pepper, salt, black pepper, and sesame oil.

Cook for 6 minutes, tossing halfway through the cooking time.

Serve and enjoy!

Beer Battered Vidalia Rings

Prep + Cook Time: 30 minutes

4 Servings

INGREDIENTS

½ pound Vidalia onions, sliced into rings

½ cup all-purpose flour

¼ cup cornmeal

½ teaspoon baking powder

Sea salt and freshly cracked black pepper, to taste

¼ teaspoon garlic powder

2 eggs, beaten

½ cup lager-style beer

1 cup plain breadcrumbs

2 tablespoons peanut oil

DIRECTIONS

Place the onion rings in the bowl with icy cold water; let them soak approximately 20 minutes; drain the onion rings and pat them dry.

In a shallow bowl, mix the flour, cornmeal, baking powder, salt, and black pepper.

Add the garlic powder, eggs and beer; mix well to combine.

In another shallow bowl, mix the breadcrumbs with the peanut oil.

Dip the onion rings in the flour/egg mixture; then, dredge in the breadcrumb mixture.

Roll to coat them evenly.

Spritz the Air Fryer basket with cooking spray; arrange the breaded onion rings in the basket.

Cook in the preheated Air Fryer at 400 degrees F for 4 to 5 minutes, turning them over halfway through the cooking time.

Enjoy!

Avocado Fries with Lime Sauce

Prep + Cook Time: 15 minutes

4 Servings

INGREDIENTS

½ cup plain flour

½ milk

½ cup tortilla chips, crushed

½ teaspoon red pepper flakes, crushed

Sea salt and ground black pepper, to taste

2 avocados, peeled, pitted and sliced

½ cup Greek yogurt

4 tablespoons mayonnaise

1 teaspoon fresh lime juice

½ teaspoon lime chili seasoning salt

DIRECTIONS

Mix the plain flour and milk in a plate.

Add the crushed tortilla chips, red pepper flakes, salt and black pepper to another rimmed plate.

Dredge the avocado slices in the flour mixture and then, coat them in the crushed tortilla chips.

Cook the avocado at 390 degrees F for about 8 minutes, shaking the basket halfway through the cooking time.

In the meantime, mix the remaining ingredients, until well combined.

Serve warm avocado fries with the lime sauce.

Enjoy!

Kale Chips with Tahini Sauce

Prep + Cook Time: 15 minutes

4 Servings

INGREDIENTS

5 cups kale leaves, torn into 1-inch pieces

1 ½ tablespoons sesame oil

½ teaspoon shallot powder

1 teaspoon garlic powder

¼ teaspoon porcini powder

½ teaspoon mustard seeds

1 teaspoon salt

⅓ cup tahini sesame butter

1 tablespoon fresh lemon juice

2 cloves garlic, minced

DIRECTIONS

Toss the kale with the sesame oil and seasonings.

Bake in the preheated Air Fryer at 350 degrees F for 10 minutes, shaking the cooking basket occasionally.

Bake until the edges are brown.

Work in batches. Meanwhile, make the sauce by whisking all ingredients in a small mixing bowl.

Serve and enjoy!

Thyme-Roasted Sweet Potatoes

Prep + Cook Time: 35 minutes

3 Servings

INGREDIENTS

1 pound sweet potatoes, peeled, cut into bite-sized pieces

2 tablespoons olive oil

1 teaspoon sea salt

¼ teaspoon freshly ground black pepper

½ teaspoon cayenne pepper

2 fresh thyme sprigs

DIRECTIONS

Arrange the potato slices in a single layer in the lightly greased cooking basket.

Add the olive oil, salt, black pepper, and cayenne pepper; toss to coat.

Bake at 380 degrees F for 30 minutes, shaking the cooking basket occasionally.

Bake until tender and slightly browned, working in batches.

Serve warm, garnished with thyme sprigs.

Cocktail Cranberry Meatballs

Prep + Cook Time: 15 minutes

5 Servings

INGREDIENTS

½ pound ground beef

½ pound ground turkey

¼ cup Parmesan cheese, grated

¼ cup breadcrumbs

1 small shallot, chopped

2 eggs, whisked

½ teaspoon garlic powder

½ teaspoon porcini powder

Sea salt and ground black pepper, to taste

1 teaspoon red pepper flakes, crushed

1 tablespoon soy sauce

1 8-ounce can jellied cranberry sauce

6 ounces tomato-based chili sauce

DIRECTIONS

In a mixing bowl, combine the ground meat together with the cheese, breadcrumbs, shallot, eggs, and spices.

Shape the mixture into 1-inch balls.

Cook the meatballs in the preheated Air Fryer at 380 degrees for 5 minutes.

Shake halfway through the cooking time.

Work in batches.

Whisk the soy sauce, cranberry sauce, and chili sauce in a mixing bowl.

Pour the sauce over the meatballs and bake an additional 2 minutes.

Serve with cocktail sticks.

Enjoy!

Teriyaki Chicken Drumettes

Prep + Cook Time: 40 minutes.

6 Servings

INGREDIENTS

1 ½ pounds chicken drumettes

Sea salt and cracked black pepper, to taste

2 tablespoons fresh chives, roughly chopped

Teriyaki Sauce:

1 tablespoon sesame oil

¼ cup soy sauce

½ cup water

¼ cup honey

½ teaspoon Five-spice powder

2 tablespoons rice wine vinegar

½ teaspoon fresh ginger, grated

2 cloves garlic, crushed

1 tablespoon corn starch dissolved in 3 tablespoons of water

DIRECTIONS

Start by preheating your Air Fryer to 380 degrees F.

Rub the chicken drumettes with salt and cracked black pepper.

Cook in the preheated Air Fryer approximately 15 minutes.

Turn them over and cook an additional 7 minutes.

While the chicken drumettes are roasting, combine the sesame oil, soy sauce, water, honey, Five-spice powder, vinegar, ginger, and garlic in a pan over medium heat.

Cook for 5 minutes, stirring occasionally.

Add the cornstarch slurry, reduce the heat, and let it simmer until the glaze thickens.

After that, brush the glaze all over the chicken drumettes.

Air-fry for a further 6 minutes or until the surface is crispy.

Serve topped with the remaining glaze and garnished with fresh chives.

Enjoy!

Blue Cheesy Potato Wedges

Prep + Cook Time: 20 minutes

4 Servings

INGREDIENTS

2Yukon Gold potatoes, peeled and cut into wedges

2 tablespoons ranch seasoning

Kosher salt, to taste

½ cup blue cheese, crumbled

DIRECTIONS

Sprinkle the potato wedges with the ranch seasoning and salt.

Grease generously the Air Fryer basket.

Place the potatoes in the cooking basket.

Roast in the preheated Air Fryer at 400 degrees for 12 minutes.

Top with the cheese and roast an additional 3 minutes or until cheese begins to melt.

Serve and enjoy!

Yakitori Japanese Chicken Skewers

Prep + Cook Time: 15 minutes

4 Servings

INGREDIENTS

½ pound chicken tenders, cut bite-sized pieces

1 clove garlic, minced

1 teaspoon coriander seeds

Sea salt and ground pepper, to taste

2 tablespoons Shoyu sauce

2 tablespoons sake

1 tablespoon fresh lemon juice

1 teaspoon sesame oil

DIRECTIONS

Place the chicken tenders, garlic, coriander, salt, black pepper, Shoyu sauce, sake, and lemon juice in a ceramic dish; cover and let it marinate for 2 hours.

Then, discard the marinade and tread the chicken tenders onto bamboo skewers.

Place the skewered chicken in the lightly greased Air Fryer basket.

Drizzle sesame oil all over the skewered chicken.

Cook at 360 degrees for 6 minutes.

Turn the skewered chicken over; brush with the reserved marinade and cook for a further 6 minutes.

Enjoy!

Pecorino Romano Meatballs

Prep + Cook Time: 15 minutes

2 Servings

INGREDIENTS

½ pound ground turkey

2 tablespoons tomato ketchup

1 teaspoon stone-ground mustard

2 tablespoons scallions, chopped

1 garlic clove, minced

¼ Pecorino-Romano cheese, grated

1 egg, beaten

½ teaspoon red pepper flakes, crushed

Sea salt and ground black pepper, to taste

DIRECTIONS

In a mixing bowl, thoroughly combine all ingredients.

Shape the mixture into 6 equal meatballs.

Transfer the meatballs to the Air Fryer cooking basket that is previously greased with a nonstick cooking spray.

Cook the meatballs at 360 degrees F for 10 to 11 minutes, shaking the basket occasionally to ensure even cooking.

An instant thermometer should read 165 degrees F and serve

Romano Cheese and Broccoli Balls

Prep + Cook Time: 25 minutes

4 Servings

INGREDIENTS

½ pound broccoli

½ cup Romano cheese, grated

2 garlic cloves, minced

1 shallot, chopped

4 eggs, beaten

2 tablespoons butter, at room temperature

½ teaspoon paprika

¼ teaspoon dried basil

Sea salt and ground black pepper, to taste

DIRECTIONS

Add the broccoli to your food processor and pulse until the consistency resembles rice.

Stir in the remaining ingredients; mix until everything is well combined.

Shape the mixture into bite-sized balls and transfer them to the lightly greased cooking basket.

Cook in the preheated Air Fryer at 375 degrees F for 16 minutes, shaking halfway through the cooking time.

Serve with cocktail sticks and tomato ketchup on the side.

Paprika and Cheese French Fries

Prep + Cook Time: 15 minutes

2 Servings

INGREDIENTS

8 ounces French fries, frozen

½ cup Monterey-Jack cheese, grated

1 teaspoon paprika

Sea salt, to taste

DIRECTIONS

Cook the French fries in your Air Fryer at 400 degrees F for about 7 minutes.

Shake the basket and continue to cook for a further 6 minutes.

Top the French fries with cheese, paprika and salt cheese.

Continue to cook for 1 minute more or until the cheese has melted.

Serve warm and enjoy!

Hot Cheesy Mushrooms Bites

Prep + Cook Time: 10 minutes

3 Servings

INGREDIENTS

1 teaspoon butter, melted

1 teaspoon fresh garlic, finely minced

4 ounces cheddar cheese, grated

4 tablespoons tortilla chips, crushed

1 tablespoon fresh coriander, chopped

½ teaspoon hot sauce

12 button mushrooms, stalks removed and chopped

Sea salt and ground black pepper, to taste

DIRECTIONS

In a mixing bowl, thoroughly combine the butter, garlic, cheddar cheese, tortilla chips, coriander, hot sauce and chopped mushrooms.

Divide the filling among mushroom caps and transfer them to the air Fryer cooking basket; season them with salt and black pepper.

Cook your mushrooms in the preheated Air Fryer at 400 degrees F for 5 minutes.

Transfer the warm mushrooms to a serving platter and serve at room temperature.

Serve and enjoy!

Pork Crackling with Sriracha Dip

Prep + Cook Time: 40 minutes

3 Servings

 INGREDIENTS

½ pound pork rind

Sea salt and ground black pepper, to taste

½ cup tomato sauce

1 teaspoon Sriracha sauce

½ teaspoon stone-ground mustard

DIRECTIONS

Rub sea salt and pepper on the skin side of the pork rind.

Allow it to sit for 30 minutes.

Then, cut the pork rind into chunks using kitchen scissors.

Roast the pork rind at 380 degrees F for 8 minutes; turn them over and cook for a further 8 minutes or until blistered.

Meanwhile, mix the tomato sauce with the Sriracha sauce and mustard.

Serve the pork crackling with the Sriracha dip and enjoy!

Cheesy Potato Puffs

Prep + Cook Time: 15 minutes

4 Servings

INGREDIENTS

8 ounces potato puffs

1 teaspoon olive oil

4 ounces cheddar cheese, shredded

½ cup tomato sauce

1 teaspoon Dijon mustard

½ teaspoon Italian seasoning mix

DIRECTIONS

Brush the potato puffs with olive oil and transfer them to the Air Fryer cooking basket.

Cook the potato puffs at 400 degrees F for 10 minutes, shaking the basket occasionally to ensure even browning.

Top them with cheese and continue to cook for 2 minutes more until the cheese melts.

Meanwhile, whisk the tomato sauce with the mustard and Italian seasoning mix.

Serve the warm potato puffs with cocktail sticks and the sauce on the side.

Serve warm.

Pepper and Bacon Mini Skewers

Prep + Cook Time: 10 minutes

4 Servings

INGREDIENTS

4 ounces bacon, diced

2 bell peppers, sliced

¼ cup barbecue sauce

1 teaspoon Ranch seasoning blend

½ cup tomato sauce

1 teaspoon jalapeno, minced

DIRECTIONS

Assemble the skewers alternating bacon and bell pepper.

Toss them with barbecue sauce and Ranch seasoning blend.

Cook the mini skewers in the preheated Air Fryer at 400 degrees F for 6 minutes.

Mix the tomato sauce and minced jalapeno.

Bon appétit!

Wonton Sausage Appetizers

Prep + Cook Time: 20 minutes

5 Servings

INGREDIENTS

½ pound ground sausage

2 tablespoons scallions, chopped

1 garlic clove, minced

½ tablespoon fish sauce

1 teaspoon Sriracha sauce

20 wonton wrappers

1 egg, whisked with 1 tablespoon water

DIRECTIONS

In a mixing bowl, thoroughly combine the ground sausage, scallions, garlic, fish sauce, and Sriracha.

Divide the mixture between the wonton wrappers.

Dip your fingers in the egg wash Fold the wonton in half.

Bring up the 2 ends of the wonton and use the egg wash to stick them together.

Pinch the edges and coat each wonton with the egg wash.

Place the folded wontons in the lightly greased cooking basket.

Cook at 360 degrees F for 10 minutes.

Work in batches and serve warm.

Serve warm.

Southwestern Caprese Bites

Prep + Cook Time: 10 minutes

2 Servings

INGREDIENTS

½ pound cherry tomatoes

1 tablespoon extra-virgin olive oil

½ pound bocconcini, drained

2 tablespoon fresh basil leaves

½ teaspoon chili powder

½ teaspoon ground cumin

¼ teaspoon garlic powder

Sea salt and ground black pepper, to taste

DIRECTIONS

Brush the cherry tomatoes with olive oil and transfer them to the cooking basket.

Bake the cherry tomatoes at 400 degrees F for 4 minutes.

Assemble the bites by using a toothpick and skewer cherry tomatoes, bocconcini and fresh basil leaves.

Season with chili powder, cumin, garlic powder, salt and black pepper.

Arrange on a nice serving platter Serve and enjoy!

Salmon, Cheese and Cucumber Bites

Prep + Cook Time: 15 minutes

3 Servings

INGREDIENTS

½ pound salmon

1 teaspoon extra-virgin olive oil

½ teaspoon onion powder

¼ teaspoon cumin powder

1 teaspoon granulated garlic

Sea salt and ground black pepper, to taste

2 ounces cream cheese

1 English cucumber, cut into 1- inch rounds

DIRECTIONS

Pat the salmon dry and drizzle it with olive oil.

Season the salmon with onion powder, cumin, granulated garlic, salt and black pepper.

Transfer the salmon to the Air Fryer cooking basket.

Cook the salmon at 400 degrees F for 5 minutes; turn the salmon over and continue to cook for 5 minutes more or until opaque.

Cut the salmon into bite- sized pieces.

Spread 1 teaspoon of cream cheese on top of each cucumber slice; top each slice with a piece of salmon.

Insert a tiny party fork down the center to keep in place.

Enjoy!

Mint Plantain Bites

Prep + Cook Time: 10 minutes

3 Servings

INGREDIENTS

1 pound plantains, peeled and cut into rounds

1 teaspoon coconut oil

A pinch of coarse sea salt

1 tablespoon mint leaves, chopped

DIRECTIONS

Start by preheating your Air Fryer to 350 degrees F.

Brush the plantain rounds with coconut oil and sprinkle with coarse sea salt.

Cook the plantain rounds in the preheated Air Fryer for 5 minutes; shake the basket and cook for a further 5 minutes or until golden on the top.

Garnish with roughly chopped mint and serve.

Enjoy!

Paprika Potato Chips

Prep + Cook Time: 50 minutes

3 Servings

INGREDIENTS

3 potatoes, thinly sliced

1 teaspoon sea salt

1 teaspoon garlic powder

1 teaspoon paprika

¼ cup ketchup

Directions

Add the sliced potatoes to a bowl with salted water.

Let them soak for 30 minutes.

Drain and rinse your potatoes.

Pat dry and toss with salt.

Cook in the preheated Air Fryer at 400 degrees F for 15 minutes, shaking the basket occasionally.

Work in batches.

Toss with the garlic powder and paprika.

Serve with ketchup.

Enjoy!

Sticky Glazed Wings

Prep + Cook Time: 30 minutes

2 Servings

INGREDIENTS

½ pound chicken wings

1 tablespoon sesame oil

2 tablespoons brown sugar

1 tablespoon Worcestershire sauce

1 tablespoon hot sauce

1 tablespoon balsamic vinegar

DIRECTIONS

Brush the chicken wings with sesame oil and transfer them to the Air Fryer cooking basket.

Cook the chicken wings at 370 degrees F for 12 minutes; turn them over and cook for a further 10 minutes.

Meanwhile, bring the other ingredients to a boil in a saucepan; cook for 2 to 3 minutes or until thoroughly cooked.

Toss the warm chicken wings with the sauce and place them on a serving platter.

Serve and enjoy!

Asian Twist Chicken Wings

Prep + Cook Time: 20 minutes

6 Servings

INGREDIENTS

1 ½ pounds chicken wings

2 teaspoons sesame oil

Kosher salt and ground black pepper, to taste

2 tablespoons tamari sauce

1 tablespoon rice vinegar

2 garlic clove, minced

2 tablespoons honey

2 sun-dried tomatoes, minced

DIRECTIONS

Toss the chicken wings with the sesame oil, salt, and pepper.

Add chicken wings to a lightly greased baking pan.

Roast the chicken wings in the preheated Air Fryer at 390 degrees F for 7 minutes.

Turn them over once or twice to ensure even cooking.

In a mixing dish, thoroughly combine the tamari sauce, vinegar, garlic, honey, and sun-dried tomatoes.

Pour the sauce all over the chicken wings; bake an additional 5 minutes.

Serve warm.

Beer-Battered Vidalia Onion Rings

Prep + Cook Time: 15 minutes

2 Servings

INGREDIENTS

½ cup all-purpose flour

½ teaspoon baking powder

¼ teaspoon cayenne pepper

¼ teaspoon dried oregano

Kosher salt and ground black pepper, to taste

1 large egg, beaten

¼ cup beer 1 cup crushed tortilla chips

½ pound Vidalia onions, cut into rings

DIRECTIONS

In a mixing bowl, thoroughly combine the flour, baking powder, cayenne pepper, oregano, salt, black pepper, egg and beer; mix to combine well.

In another shallow bowl, place the crushed tortilla chips.

Dip the Vidalia rings in the beer mixture; then, coat the rings with the crushed tortilla chips, pressing to adhere.

Transfer the onion rings to the Air Fryer cooking basket and spritz them with a nonstick spray.

Cook the onion rings at 380 degrees F for about 8 minutes, shaking the basket halfway through the cooking time to ensure even browning.

Serve and enjoy!

Coconut Banana Chips

Prep + Cook Time: 10 minutes

2 Servings

INGREDIENTS

1 large banana, peeled and sliced 1 teaspoon coconut oil

¼ teaspoon ground cinnamon

A pinch of coarse salt

2 tablespoons coconut flakes

DIRECTIONS

Toss the banana slices with the coconut oil, cinnamon and salt.

Transfer banana slices to the Air Fryer cooking basket.

Cook the banana slices at 375 degrees F for about 8 minutes, shaking the basket every 2 minutes.

Scatter coconut flakes over the banana slices and let banana chips cool slightly before serving.

Enjoy!

Eggplant Parm Chips

Prep + Cook Time: 30 minutes

2 Servings

INGREDIENTS

½ pound eggplant, cut into rounds

Kosher salt and ground black pepper, to taste

½ teaspoon shallot powder

½ teaspoon porcini powder

½ teaspoon garlic powder

¼ teaspoon cayenne pepper

½ cup Parmesan cheese, grated

DIRECTIONS

Toss the eggplant rounds with the remaining ingredients until well coated on both sides.

Bake the eggplant chips at 400 degrees F for 15 minutes; shake the basket and continue to cook for 15 minutes more.

Let cool slightly, eggplant chips will crisp up as it cools. Enjoy!

Mexican Crunchy Cheese Straws

Prep + Cook Time: 15 minutes

3 Servings

INGREDIENTS

½ cup almond flour

¼ teaspoon xanthan gum

¼ teaspoon shallot powder

¼ teaspoon garlic powder

¼ teaspoon ground cumin

1 egg yolk, whisked

1 ounce Manchego cheese, grated

2 ounces Cotija cheese, grated

DIRECTIONS

Mix all ingredients until everything is well incorporated.

Twist the batter into straw strips and place them on a baking mat inside your Air Fryer.

Cook the cheese straws in your Air Fryer at 360 degrees F for 5 minutes; turn them over and cook an additional 5 minutes.

Let the cheese straws cool before serving.

Enjoy!

Greek-Style Deviled Eggs

Prep + Cook Time: 20 minutes

2 Servings

INGREDIENTS

eggs

1 tablespoon chives, chopped

1 tablespoon parsley, chopped

2 tablespoons Kalamata olives, pitted and chopped

1 tablespoon Greek-style yogurt

1 teaspoon habanero pepper, seeded and chopped

Sea salt and crushed red pepper flakes, to taste

DIRECTIONS

Place the wire rack in the Air Fryer basket and lower the eggs onto the rack.

Cook the eggs at 260 degrees F for 15 minutes.

Transfer the eggs to an ice-cold water bath to stop cooking.

Peel the eggs under cold running water; slice them into halves, separating the whites and yolks.

Mash the egg yolks with the remaining ingredients and mix to combine.

Spoon the yolk mixture into the egg whites and serve well chilled.

Enjoy!

Puerto Rican Tostones

Prep + Cook Time: 15 minutes

2 Servings

INGREDIENTS

1 ripe plantain, sliced

1 tablespoon sunflower oil

A pinch of grated nutmeg

A pinch of kosher salt

DIRECTIONS

Toss the plantains with the oil, nutmeg, and salt in a bowl.

Cook in the preheated Air Fryer at 400 degrees F for 10 minutes, shaking the cooking basket halfway through the cooking time.

Adjust the seasonings to taste and serve immediately.

Green Bean Crisps

Prep + Cook Time: 20 minutes

4 Servings

INGREDIENTS

1 egg, beaten

¼ cup cornmeal

¼ cup parmesan, grated

1 teaspoon sea salt

½ teaspoon red pepper flakes, crushed

1 pound green beans

2 tablespoons grapeseed oil

DIRECTIONS

In a mixing bowl, combine together the egg, cornmeal, parmesan, salt, and red pepper flakes; mix to combine well.

Dip the green beans into the batter and transfer them to the cooking basket.

Brush with the grapeseed oil.

Cook in the preheated Air Fryer at 390 degrees F for 4 minutes.

Shake the basket and cook for a further 3 minutes.

Work in batches.

Taste, adjust the seasonings and serve.

Serve warm.

Quick and Easy Popcorn

Prep + Cook Time: 20 minutes

4 Servings

INGREDIENTS

2 tablespoons dried corn kernels

1 teaspoon safflower oil

Kosher salt, to taste

1 teaspoon red pepper flakes, crushed

DIRECTIONS

Add the dried corn kernels to the Air Fryer basket; brush with safflower oil.

Cook at 395 degrees F for 15 minutes, shaking the basket every 5 minutes.

Sprinkle with salt and red pepper flakes.

Enjoy!

Homemade Ranch Tater Tots

Prep + Cook Time: 15 minutes

2 Servings

INGREDIENTS

½ pound potatoes, peeled and shredded

½ teaspoon hot paprika

½ teaspoon dried marjoram

1 teaspoon Ranch seasoning mix

2 tablespoons Colby cheese, finely grated

about ⅓ cup 1 teaspoon butter, melted

Sea salt and ground black pepper, to taste

DIRECTIONS

In a mixing bowl, thoroughly combine all ingredients until everything is well incorporated.

Transfer your tater tots to a lightly greased Air Fryer cooking basket.

Cook your tater tots in the preheated Air Fryer at 400 degrees F for 12 minutes, shaking the basket halfway through the cooking time to ensure even browning.

Serve and enjoy!

Barbecue Little Smokies

Prep + Cook Time: 20 minutes

6 Servings

INGREDIENTS

1 pound beef cocktail wieners

10 ounces barbecue sauce

DIRECTIONS

Start by preheating your Air Fryer to 380 degrees F.

Prick holes into your sausages using a fork and transfer them to the baking pan.

Cook for 13 minutes.

Spoon the barbecue sauce into the pan and cook an additional 2 minutes.

Serve with toothpicks.

Enjoy!

Baby Carrots with Asian Flair

Prep + Cook Time: 20 minutes

3 Servings

INGREDIENTS

1 pound baby carrots

2 tablespoons sesame oil

½ teaspoon Szechuan pepper

1 teaspoon Wuxiang powder Five-spice powder

1 tablespoon honey

1 large garlic clove, crushed

1 1-inch piece fresh ginger root, peeled and grated

2 tablespoons tamari sauce

DIRECTIONS

Start by preheating your Air Fryer to 380 degrees F.

Toss all ingredients together and place them in the Air Fryer basket.

Cook for 15 minutes, shaking the basket halfway through the cooking time.

Enjoy!

Greek-Style Squash Chips

Prep + Cook Time: 25 minutes

4 Servings

INGREDIENTS

½ cup seasoned breadcrumbs

½ cup Parmesan cheese, grated

Sea salt and ground black pepper, to taste

¼ teaspoon oregano

2 yellow squash, cut into slices

2 tablespoons grapeseed oil

Sauce:

½ cup Greek-style yogurt

1 tablespoon fresh cilantro, chopped

1 garlic clove, minced Freshly ground black pepper, to your liking

DIRECTIONS

In a shallow bowl, thoroughly combine the seasoned breadcrumbs, Parmesan, salt, black pepper, and oregano.

Dip the yellow squash slices in the prepared batter, pressing to adhere.

Brush with the grapeseed oil and cook in the preheated Air Fryer at 400 degrees F for 12 minutes.

Shake the Air Fryer basket periodically to ensure even cooking.

Work in batches.

While the chips are baking, whisk the sauce ingredients; place in your refrigerator until ready to serve.

Enjoy!

Cajun Cheese Sticks

Prep + Cook Time: 15 minutes

4 Servings

INGREDIENTS

½ cup all-purpose flour

2 eggs

½ cup parmesan cheese, grated

1 tablespoon Cajun seasonings

8 cheese sticks, kid- friendly

¼ cup ketchup

DIRECTIONS

To begin, set up your breading station.

Place the all-purpose flour in a shallow dish.

In a separate dish, whisk the eggs.

Finally, mix the parmesan cheese and Cajun seasoning in a third dish.

Start by dredging the cheese sticks in the flour; then, dip them into the egg.

Press the cheese sticks into the parmesan mixture, coating evenly.

Place the breaded cheese sticks in the lightly greased Air Fryer basket.

Cook at 380 degrees F for 6 minutes.

Serve with ketchup and enjoy!

Kale Chips with White Horseradish Mayo

Prep + Cook Time: 10 minutes

1 Servings

INGREDIENTS

2 cups loosely packed kale

1 teaspoon sesame oil

Sea salt and ground black pepper, to taste

1 teaspoon sesame seeds, lightly toasted

1 ounce mayonnaise

1 teaspoon prepared white horseradish

DIRECTIONS

Toss the kale pieces with sesame oil, salt and black pepper.

Cook the kale pieces at 370 degrees F for 2 minutes; shake the basket and continue to cook for 2 minutes more.

Meanwhile, make the horseradish mayo by whisking the mayonnaise and prepared horseradish.

Let cool slightly, kale chips will crisp up as it cools.

Sprinkle toasted sesame seeds over the kale chips.

Serve the kale chips with the horseradish mayo.

Enjoy!

Mexican Cheesy Zucchini Bites

Prep + Cook Time: 25 minutes

4 Servings

INGREDIENTS

1 large-sized zucchini, thinly sliced

½ cup flour

¼ cup yellow cornmeal

1 egg, whisked

½ cup tortilla chips, crushed

½ cup Queso Añejo, grated

Salt and cracked pepper, to taste

DIRECTIONS

Pat dry the zucchini slices with a kitchen towel.

Mix the remaining ingredients in a shallow bowl; mix until everything is well combined.

Dip each zucchini slice in the prepared batter.

Cook in the preheated Air Fryer at 400 degrees F for 12 minutes, shaking the basket halfway through the cooking time.

Work in batches until the zucchini slices are crispy and golden brown.

Enjoy!

Homemade Apple Chips

Prep + Cook Time: 20 minutes

4 Servings

INGREDIENTS

2 cooking apples, cored and thinly sliced

1 teaspoon peanut oil

¼ teaspoon ground cloves

¼ teaspoon ground cinnamon

1 tablespoon smooth peanut butter

DIRECTIONS

Toss the apple slices with the peanut oil.

Bake at 350 degrees F for 5 minutes; shake the basket to ensure even cooking and continue to cook an additional 5 minutes.

Spread each apple slice with a little peanut butter and sprinkle with ground cloves and cinnamon.

Serve and enjoy!

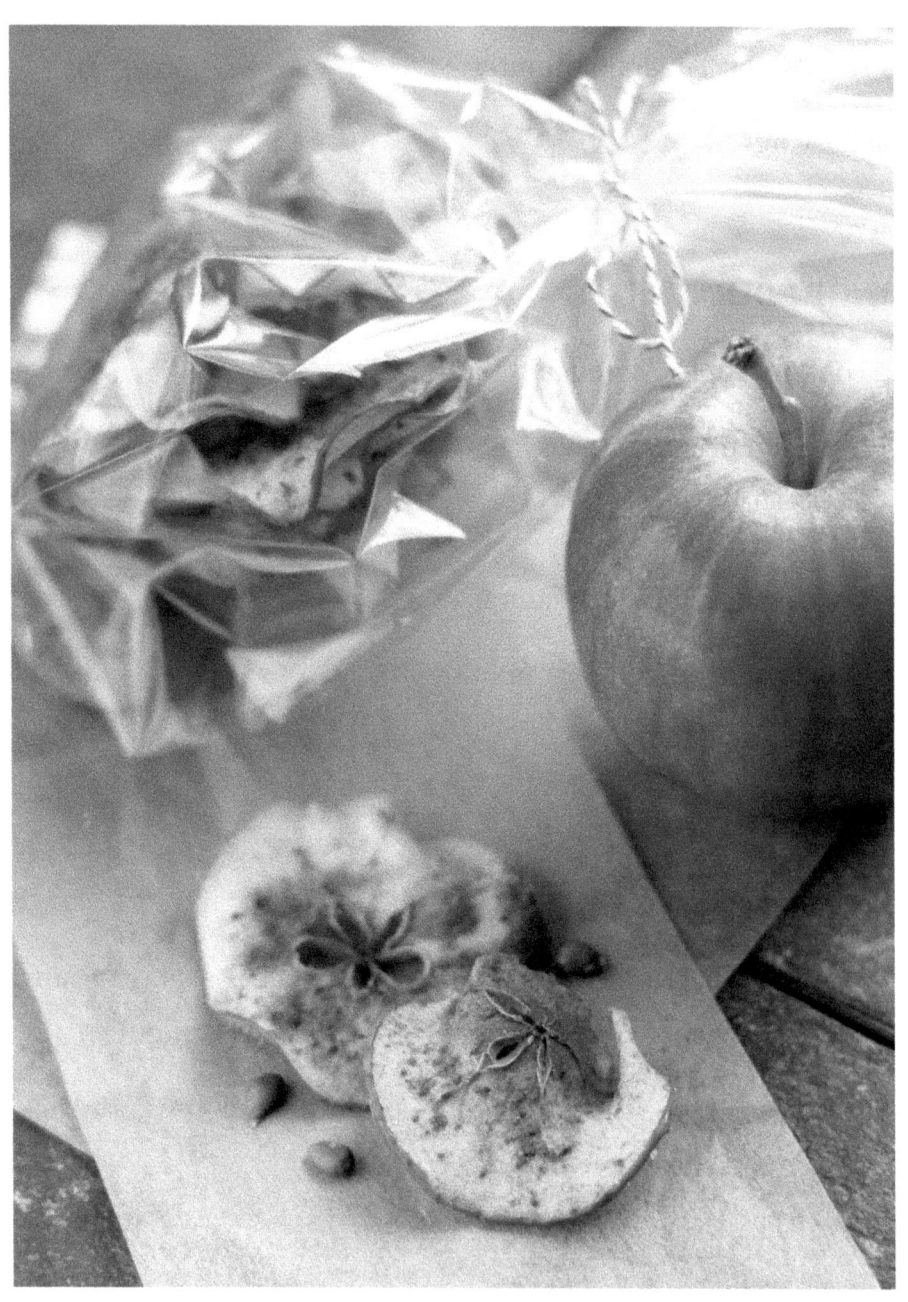

Easy and Delicious Pizza Puffs

Prep + Cook Time: 15 minutes

6 Servings

INGREDIENTS

6 ounces crescent roll dough

½ cup mozzarella cheese, shredded

3 ounces pepperoni

3 ounces mushrooms, chopped

1 teaspoon oregano

1 teaspoon garlic powder

¼ cup Marina sauce, for dipping

DIRECTIONS

Unroll the crescent dough.

Roll out the dough using a rolling pin; cut into 6 pieces.

Place the cheese, pepperoni, and mushrooms in the center of each pizza puff.

Sprinkle with oregano and garlic powder.

Fold each corner over the filling using wet hands.

Press together to cover the filling entirely and seal the edges.

Now, spritz the bottom of the Air Fryer basket with cooking oil.

Lay the pizza puffs in a single layer in the cooking basket.

Work in batches.

Bake at 370 degrees F for 5 to 6 minutes or until golden brown.

Serve with the marinara sauce for dipping.

Party Greek Keftedes

Prep + Cook Time: 20 minutes

6 Servings

INGREDIENTS

Greek Keftedes:

½ pound mushrooms, chopped

½ pound pork sausage, chopped

1 teaspoon shallot powder

1 teaspoon granulated garlic

1 teaspoon dried rosemary

1 teaspoon dried basil

1 teaspoon dried oregano

2 eggs

2 tablespoons cornbread crumbs

Tzatziki Dip:

1 Lebanese cucumbers, grated, juice squeezed out

1 cup full-fat Greek yogurt

1 tablespoon fresh lemon juice

1 garlic clove, minced

1 tablespoon extra-virgin olive oil

½ teaspoon salt

DIRECTIONS

In a mixing bowl, thoroughly combine all ingredients for the Greek keftedes.

Shape the meat mixture into bite-sized balls.

Cook in the preheated Air Fryer at 380 degrees for 10 minutes, shaking the cooking basket once or twice to ensure even cooking.

Meanwhile, make the tzatziki dip by mixing all ingredients.

Serve the keftedes with cocktail sticks and tzatziki dip on the side.

Enjoy!

Three Meat Cheesy Omelet

Prep + Cook Time: 20 minutes

2 Servings

INGREDIENTS

1 beef sausage, chopped

4 slices prosciutto, chopped

3 oz salami, chopped

1 cup mozzarella cheese, grated

4 eggs

1 green onion, chopped

1 tbsp ketchup

1 tsp fresh parsley, chopped

DIRECTIONS

Preheat air fryer to 350 F.

Whisk the eggs with ketchup in a bowl.

Stir in green onion, mozzarella, salami, and prosciutto.

AirFry the sausage in a greased baking tray in the fryer for 2 minutes.

Slide-out and pour the egg mixture on top.

Cook for another 8 minutes until golden.

Serve sliced with parsley.

Orange Creamy Cupcakes

Prep + Cook Time: 25 minutes

4 Servings

INGREDIENTS

Lemon Frosting:

1 cup plain yogurt

2 tbsp sugar

1 orange, juiced

1 tbsp orange zest

7 oz cream cheese

Cake:

2 lemons, seeded and quartered

½ cup flour + extra for basing

¼ tsp salt

2 tbsp sugar1 tsp baking powder

1 tsp vanilla extract

2 eggs

½ cup butter, softened

2 tbsp milk

DIRECTIONS

In a bowl, add yogurt and cream cheese and mix until smooth.

Add in orange juice and zest and whisk well.

Gradually add the sugar and stir until smooth.

Make sure the frost is not runny.

Set aside.

Place the lemon quarters in a food processor and process until pureed.

Add in the flour, baking powder, softened butter, milk, eggs, vanilla extract, sugar, and salt.

Process again until smooth. Preheat air fryer to 360 F.

Flour the bottom of 4 cupcake cases and spoon the batter into the cases, ¾ way up.

Place them in the air fryer and bake for 12 minutes or until the inserted toothpick comes out clean.

Once ready, remove and let cool.

Design the cupcakes with the frosting and serve.

Avocado Tempura

Prep + Cook Time: 10 minutes

4 Servings

INGREDIENTS

½ cup breadcrumbs

½ tsp salt

1 avocado, pitted, peeled, and sliced

½ cup liquid from beans

DIRECTIONS

Preheat air fryer to 360 F.

In a bowl, add the crumbs and salt and mix to combine.

Sprinkle the avocado with the beans' liquid and then coat in the crumbs.

Arrange the slices in one layer inside the fryer and AirFry for 8-10 minutes, shaking once or twice.

Serve warm

Blueberry Oat Bars

Prep + Cook Time: 20 minutes

12 bars

INGREDIENTS

1 cups rolled oats

¼ cup ground almonds

¼ cup sugar

1 tsp baking powder

½ tsp ground cinnamon

2 eggs, lightly beaten

½ cup canola oil

½ cup milk

1 tsp vanilla extract

2 cups blueberries

DIRECTIONS

Spray a baking pan that fits in your air fryer with cooking spray.

In a bowl, add oats, almonds, sugar, baking powder, and cinnamon and stir well.

In another bowl, whisk eggs, canola oil, milk, and vanilla.

Stir the wet ingredients gently into the oat mixture.

Fold in the blueberries.

Pour the mixture into the pan and place it in the fryer.

Cook for 10 minutes at 350 F.

Let it cool on a wire rack.

Cut into 12 bars.

www.ingramcontent.com/pod-product-compliance
Lightning Source LLC
Chambersburg PA
CBHW071110030426
42336CB00013BA/2025